The Chiropractor Hoax

The True Story of Chiropractic Medicine You've Never Been Told

By John Morrison

Publisher: ZML Corp LLC
ISBN: 9781797011080

TABLE OF CONTENTS

DISCLAIMER

This book is written for informational and entertainment purposes only. The author is not a medical doctor or chiropractic physician, nor is he affiliated with any medical doctors or chiropractic physicians. This book is copyrighted 2019 all rights reserved, published by ZML Corp LLC. It is illegal to copy or reproduce this book without written consent from the author or publisher.

John Morrison

Introduction

We've all heard the claims, "go to a chiropractor, they'll help with your back pain." Or maybe we have a friend who swears by their chiropractor for fixing their back or neck pain. Maybe you've gone to a chiropractor yourself, but didn't really know if they helped you or not. I mean they're a doctor, so they have to know something about your health right?

Hi, my name is John Morrison and in this book, I'll be teaching you about chiropractic medicine. We will start at the rocky beginnings, with the one man who started it all, and progress to what it has evolved into today. I will go over the science behind chiropractics and case studies comparing chiropractic therapy to conventional modern medicine. And after all is said and done, I will have proved to you that chiropractic medicine, and I use the word medicine very loosely here, is nothing more than a sham with no scientific basis, which takes billions of dollars each year from unknowing clients, similar to many other forms of unproven alternative medicines. And while there are minimal risk with other forms of alternative medicine, chiropractic medicine risks patients short and long term health, and can potentially even cause death. So hang on to your walker, we're about to take a ride into the wild, unheard of side of the chiropractic medicine. Yeeeee haaaa!

CHAPTER 1
My Experience With Chiropractors

Like many of you reading this book, you may have already been to a chiropractor. If you haven't that's even better, I'm saving you time, money, and potential health problems. My first experience with a chiropractor was to help cure a sinus issue I was experiencing. Chiropractic websites described this as an issue affecting the spine and neck, and was something that could be treated with chiropractic intervention. I lived in South Carolina, United States at the time and found a local chiropractor in my area who, to my surprise, was covered by my health insurance! I was surprised because I thought it was considered alternative medicine, yet my insurance believed it could improve my health enough to cover it (I'll explain why they do this later in the book).

When I went into the chiropractor's office, it was quite impressive. He had his doctorate hanging on the wall stating he was a board certified chiropractic physician and was thus considered a doctor. He talked with me about my ailments, past medical history, and while making no guarantees, he told me my condition would most likely improve with his adjustments. After placing me on his table and going over my back with his hands, as well as giving my neck a few turns, he stated that my neck was out of alignment. He said that putting it back into alignment would take many treatments, as the body will naturally want to go back to its original position. I agreed and we started therapy. Before I knew it, I was a villain in a Bruce Lee movie. The chiropractor gently placed his hands over my chin and the back of my skull and... CRACK, spun my neck in what felt like a 90 degrees sideways motion. He then spun it the other way 90 degrees and... CRACK. He performed a few minor adjustments on my lower back, and then sent me to his secretary to schedule a follow up appointment. I ended up going four times over the course of two weeks, and each time the chiropractor performed the same neck manipulation technique on me, as well as providing minor adjustments to my back. After the fourth treatment I decided it wasn't working and stopped going.

Fast forward a couple years, and I'm now living in North Carolina, United States. At this time I was still experiencing my sinus issues and decided to give chiropractics another try. I found a chiropractor in my area and went in for a free consultation. Because it was my first time there, the chiropractic physician stated he needed an x-ray of my entire back and neck. While I understood it was maybe needed for the provider to get a better view of what my bones looked like, I was a little hesitant because of the radiation factor. Here you have an x-ray taken of your entire spine, which exposes you to much more radiation than a small wrist x-ray you may get at a primary doctor's office. Not only this, primary care doctors offer lead shields to help protect vital organs from radiation; this was not the case at the chiropractor. Knowing all this, I declined the x-ray. Next his assistant slowly rolled a device down my neck and spine called the "MyoVision Scanner 8000." They told me this device could detect any nerves or bones out of alignment in my back, simply by passing over them. The results would then show on a computer screen and the chiropractor would be able to fix me. [1]

At this point the quack signal started flashing in my mind. Granted I'm an open minded individual, but a device that could determine the exact point in my back that was "out of alignment" just by rolling it along the spine. Why has my primary care doctor never brought up this device? Why aren't medical doctors using this device? Couldn't this device help the thousands of Americans who suffer with back pain pinpoint their issue? It just didn't make any sense to me.

I then asked the chiropractic physician if he would be treating my disorder with anything in addition to the spinal and neck manipulation, such as supplements, diet, etc. He brought up some homeopathic supplements that would be beneficial for me. At this point I decided it was time to leave. If you're unfamiliar with homeopathic medicine, it's even worse than chiropractic medicine when it comes to how disproven of a therapy it is. I'll be coming out with a book on it in the near future, but if you're unfamiliar, just know homeopathic medicine is a multi-billion dollar industry which has been proven time and time again to do absolutely nothing, and work only by the placebo effect.

So I was polite; I thanked the chiropractor for his time, thanked his assistant, and then proceeded to leave the office. This final visit to a chiropractor inspired me to start doing more research on the subject, which then inspired me to write this book. When I started writing this book, I had no idea how deep this rabbit hole would go, and how ill-equipped the chiropractic profession truly was. What I discovered about chiropractic therapy, chiropractic education, and the unknowing ignorance shared by the general public was mind blowing.

I hope to save my fellow reader the time and money lost, as well as the potential health risks associated with going to a chiropractor. And for you to learn the truth behind the profession of chiropractic medicine for your own knowledge and to share with your friends and family.

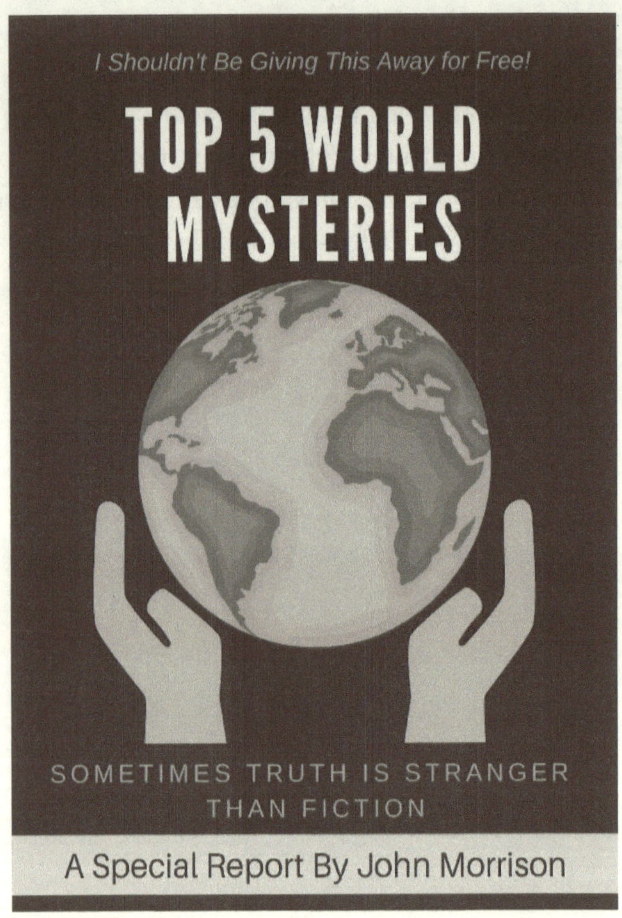

As a **token of appreciation** to my readers, I am offering my special report above titled *Top 5 World Mysteries* **absolutely free!** Just copy and paste the link below into your browser, put in your email address, and it will be immediately sent to you.

fastlink.xyz/topfive

CHAPTER 2
History of Chiropractic Medicine

I want you to brace yourself as a lot of this may be new to you, as it was for me. All along I thought chiropractors practiced alongside medical doctors, getting taught from the same medical textbooks and trainers, but this is not the case at all.

The year is 1897 and Daniel David Palmer, a known "magnetic healer" from Davenport, Iowa had a new idea. To give you a little background, magnetic healing is a pseudoscientific claim that passing a magnet over certain parts of the body can have beneficial health effects (who knew fridge magnets could be so fun). At the time, Daniel had concocted a theory that, not only were magnets beneficial, but that the back was the central healing center of the body. And as such, by adjusting the back, any part of the body could thus be healed. Daniel is famously quoted in his book from 1910 saying,

"a subluxated vertebrae . . . is the cause of 95 percent of all

I want to make you aware this was a theory with no basis in science, but instead just an abstract hypothesis from someone who was not a doctor, but a magnetic healer. Daniel claims to have been introduced to a deaf janitor whom he was able to test his new theory on. According to the legend, the deaf janitor allowed Mr. Palmer to adjust his back. A little snap, crackle, pop and the deaf janitor could now hear! A true Christmas miracle! [3]

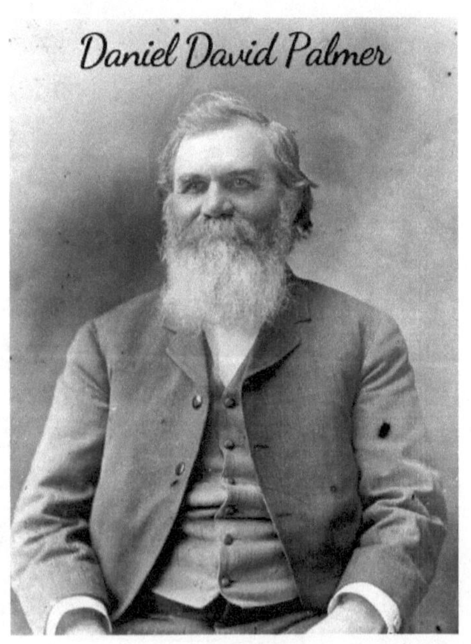

While this is the story David gives, David's daughter tells a different version of the story. She claims that her father overheard the janitor telling a joke outside a bar to a few other men. When the janitor told the punchline, out of pure laughter, David slapped the janitor on his back. A few days later, the janitor told David his hearing had improved. [4]

Whatever the true story, this is a very influential part of chiropractic history, and what began the whole profession. The story is still brought up to this day by chiropractors. Palmer felt this was enough evidence to begin expanding on his theory. He soon opened "Chiropractic Schools of Medicine," some of which still exists to this day. One example is the Palmer College of Chiropractic in Iowa, a school that accepts anyone with a semi-working pulse and wallet (which we'll get to later). During this time, Palmer states he was given instructions on more elaborate forms of chiropractic medicine from the spirit world. He reported that he obtained chiropractic instructions from the ghost of a medical doctor named Dr. Jim Atkinson. He wrote in his 1910 book:

"The knowledge and philosophy given [to] me by Dr. Jim Atkinson, an intelligent spiritual being, together with explanations of phenomena, principles resolved

from causes, effects, powers, laws and utility, appealed to my reason. The method by which I obtained an explanation of certain physical phenomena, from an intelligence in the spiritual world, is known in biblical language as inspiration. In a great measure The Chiropractor's Adjuster was written under such spiritual promptings." [2]

These instructions, from a ghost, helped him further expand on the chiropractic theory.

CHAPTER 3
The Chiropractic Theory

I want you to understand that chiropractic medicine has absolutely no basis in modern medicine. As stated, it was started by an alternative practitioner with fabricated beginnings who claimed to talk to spirits, and the science behind it has remained the same into modern times.

Chiropractic theory is based on a notion known as "vertebral subluxation." The theory purports that the body has natural healing powers located in the spinal column, and when subluxation or "misalignment" occurs in the spine, it can affect other areas of the body. There are nerves that run through the spinal column, and when one of these nerves is pinched or irritated, it can interfere with the signals sent throughout the body. It's said the nerves in each section of the spine link to different parts of the body. As such, when subluxation is corrected, this in turn will fix the part of the body which correlates with that section of the spinal column.

This is quite similar to, and may have even been

extracted from other alternative medicine treatments such as reflexology and acupuncture. Reflexology states different parts of the base of the foot connect to different parts of the body, and acupuncture states different parts of the tongue connect to organs in the body. But in summary, the theory is stating that most any ailment or condition affecting the human body can be healed by effectively restoring order in the spinal column. [5]

Here is a picture of a human spine, labeled with subluxation points, which describes the different ailments caused by misalignment of the spine:

Spinal Nerve Function
Every Cell of Your Body Has a Nerve Component

VERTEBRAL LEVEL	NERVE ROOT*	INNERVATION	POSSIBLE SYMPTOMS
C1	C1	Intracranial Blood Vessels • Eyes • Lacrimal Gland • Parotid Gland • Scalp • Base of Skull • Neck Muscles • Diaphragm	Headaches • Migraine Headaches • Dizziness • Sinus Problems • Allergies • Head Colds • Fatigue • Vision Problems • Runny Nose • Sore Throat • Stiff Neck
C2	C2		
C3	C3		
C4	C4		
C5	C5	• Neck Muscles • Shoulders • Elbows • Arms • Wrists • Hands • Fingers • Esophagus • Heart • Lungs • Chest	• Cough • Croup • Arm Pain • Hand and Finger Numbness or Tingling • Asthma • Heart Conditions • High Blood Pressure
C5	C6		
C6	C7		
C7	C8		
	T1		
T1	T2	Arms • Esophagus • Heart • Lungs • Chest • Larynx • Trachea	Wrist, Hand and Finger Numbness or Pain • Middle Back Pain • Congestion • Difficulty Breathing • Asthma • High Blood Pressure • Heart Conditions
T2	T3		
T3	T4		
T4			
T5	T5	Gallbladder • Liver • Diaphragm • Stomach • Pancreas • Spleen • Kidneys • Small Intestine • Appendix • Adrenals	• Bronchitis • Pneumonia • Gallbladder Conditions • Jaundice • Liver Conditions • Stomach Problems • Ulcers • Gastritis • Kidney Problems
T6	T6		
	T7		
T7	T8		
T8	T9		
T9	T10		
T10	T11	Small Intestines • Colon • Uterus	
T11	T12	Uterus • Colon • Buttocks	
T12			
L1	L1	Large Intestines • Buttocks • Groin • Reproductive Organs • Colon • Thighs • Knees • Legs • Feet	Constipation • Colitis • Diarrhea • Gas Pain • Irritable Bowel • Bladder Problems • Menstrual Problems • Low Back Pain • Pain or Numbness in Legs
L2	L2		
L3	L3		
L4	L4		
L4	L5		
L5			
	SACRAL	Buttocks • Reproductive Organs • Bladder • Prostate Gland • Legs • Ankles • Feet • Toes	Constipation • Diarrhea • Bladder Problems • Menstrual Problems • Lower Back Pain • Pain or Numbness in Legs

Your spine has four main regions associated with it. Going from top to bottom you have your: cervical region (neck), thoracic region (upper back), lumbar region (lower back), and sacral region (tailbone). Chiropractic theory states that if you have a heart problem, your T2, as in the 2nd disc in your thoracic region, is currently "out of alignment." And so, by adjusting the T2 area of the spine, any heart issue you are experiencing will alleviate itself. Or that by adjusting the L4 bone, your constipation will go away. Or that by adjusting the C1, your migraines will go away. If you notice in the chart above, almost any condition you can think of is labeled and reportedly curable by adjusting some part of the back. Has this ever been proven? No, however there have been quite a few studies disproving it. This is the main theory chiropractic physicians ascribe to. Why do they do this?

One reason is because they actually believe it, as it's the science taught to them in their four years of chiropractic schooling. The second reason could involve the almighty dollar, as the more conditions you can supposedly treat, the more people who will come to your clinic and give you their money. Don't think this could be the old way chiropractics was done, and things are changing to keep up with modern times. This is the currently taught theory! Here is a brief excerpt from the website of Life College West, a chiropractic school in California:

"Through chiropractic adjustments, nervous system interference due to abnormalities in the musculoskeletal relationships of the vertebrae (called subluxations) can be corrected. This allows the nervous system to function properly, enabling the

body to heal through its own natural recuperative powers. Chiropractors are highly skilled in the art of adjusting all the articulations of the body. Adjustments are gentle and specific physical maneuvers that can be applied safely to people of any age." [6]

And here is an excerpt from the Association of Chiropractic Colleges, representing a large number of schools throughout the United States and Canada:

"Chiropractic is concerned with the preservation and restoration of health, and focuses particular attention on the subluxation. A subluxation is a complex of functional and or pathological articular changes that compromise neural integrity and may influence organ system function and general health." [7]

A small number of chiropractors have begun to get away from this "spine heals all" theory of chiropractics as they understand it's not based in modern science and does not resonate well with all patients. The ones getting away from classic chiropractic theory focus strictly on patients with spine and neck pain, while getting away from curing high blood pressure by adjusting the C7 disc. While this may appear more reasonable, there is still almost no evidence that any of these adjustments help with pain. Remember, chiropractic theory teaches that "spine heals all," and by strictly adjusting parts of the spine for back pain, you are now deviating from true chiropractic medicine and creating new theories. While serious risk is low, there is evidence that adjustments can make patient's pain worse or cause long term health problems, particularly if neck adjustments are performed, which we'll get into later in the book.

Almost all chiropractors require a full spinal x-ray at your first visit, which they say is needed to evaluate what is causing your pain. This type of full body x-ray exposes you to unnecessary radiation. While real subluxations, as in dislocations of the spine would be visible on an x-ray, chiropractic subluxations are different. These supposed misalignments of the spine can be incredibly small, making them unrecognizable via x-ray. This was verified in a letter sent back to a physician (MD) who posed this question to Palmer College of Chiropractic.

"Chiropractors do not make the claim to be able to read a specific subluxation from an x-ray film.

> *[They] can read spinal distortion, which indicates the possible presence of a subluxation and can confirm the actual presence of a subluxation by other physical findings"* [8]

I would assume most chiropractors perform an x-ray because it appears to lend more credibility to whatever they say is causing your pain. They can look at your x-ray with you, point to a few spots, and "pinpoint" the issue. Considering most people have no idea how to read an x-ray, or anything about subluxation, they would just nod their head in agreeance. The only time you would need a full spinal x-ray like this would be if there was an actual possible break somewhere along your spine. And for the vast majority of chiropractic patients, this is not the case.

Many chiropractic offices offer a mix of other, equally as quacky treatment options mixed into their clinic; this includes homeopathic medicine and acupuncture. Many also offer massage therapy, which isn't quacky and could help to explain why some people feel better after visiting the chiropractor. I mean who doesn't feel good after a massage?

What you need to know about both homeopathic

medicine and acupuncture is just like chiropractics, they are not based on modern medicine and clinical trials have failed to produce evidence either are effective. Just like chiropractics, they most likely provide minor beneficial results for some patients because of the placebo effect. What matters here though is the financial benefits which the chiropractor is able to obtain. Additional forms of any "medicine" incorporated into your office means more potential customers and more potential sales. If you are a chiropractor who owns an office, you can now rent out part of your office to an acupuncturist, you can rent out another room to a massage therapist, and you can sell homeopathic medicine to each client, all of which provide additional income. People already believe what you are telling them about their back, so they will most likely trust other medical recommendations you offer. It becomes more financially beneficial to provide all these services out of your office.

CHAPTER 4
Clinical Studies

First, I want to explain the difference between clinical studies, case studies, and anecdotal evidence. Clinical studies take a group of participants ranging in number from just a few to hundreds of participants, and then perform a study on these individuals. The best clinical studies are what are called "double blind placebo controlled" studies. This is where neither the provider nor the patient know if the actual therapeutic treatment is being administered, or if a "sham treatment" or sugar pill is being administered. These studies take into account the very well-known placebo effect. For those unfamiliar, the placebo effect is a well-documented effect dating back to when it started being discovered in the early 1800's. It is when your own mind thinks it is receiving some type of beneficial treatment, and thus you feel less pain, symptoms, etc. of whatever disorder you're being treated for. In the past, they would provide subjects pills full of sugar, say it was medicine, and the subjects would report getting better. There's been studies where subjects have been given non-alcohol drinks, but told the drinks contained alcohol, and they started feeling "drunk." The mind is very powerful. This is why clinical studies must take into account the placebo effect, so they are able to determine if the actual treatment method is working, or if the patient is just experiencing placebo.

Case studies are similar to clinical studies, except they apply to a single person or single group. The researcher is able to get a more in depth analysis for their research. Many times with case studies, the participants have already reported benefits or outcomes. An example being case studies involving children who have reported memories of reincarnation, at which point researchers start conducting research on said children.

Anecdotal evidence is when you hear of a friend's dad, or possibly a co-worker, who state they visited a chiropractor and their back pain was improved. There is no research involved or study of participants. Anecdotal evidence is the least reliable form of evidence, and should be regarded as such. This is more or less hear-say, and the chiropractor could have fixed their back problems, or time could have fixed it or sleeping differently could have fixed it, and it was just a coincidence they happened to see the chiropractor around the same time. They then attributed this decrease in pain to chiropractic treatment, when in actuality it had nothing to do with the chiropractor. Or it's possible that their pain actually did improve, but it was nothing more than the placebo effect.

What I'm trying to impress upon you with these examples is anytime you hear of someone getting better with chiropractic treatment, it's anecdotal evidence, and not actually proven. There have been many clinical studies on the treatment, and the findings don't bid well for chiropractics.

In 1996, a large scale study was performed that included 8 clinical trials of chiropractic treatment for low back pain. The authors found "no convincing evidence for the effectiveness of chiropractic for acute or chronic low back pain." Some in the community stated the study was flawed in its design and execution. Since then, several other better controlled clinical trials have emerged, involving hundreds of patients. These studies "did not show an advantage of chiropractic over control treatments." Control treatment being any other treatment option other than chiropractic manipulation, with examples being steroid injections, acupuncture, and oral medication. [9]

While it already doesn't look well for chiropractic medicine, if the issues associated with these studies were fixed, it would have been even worse. The first issue is few of these studies controlled for the placebo effect. This is extremely important when evaluating any type of medical treatment. Considering the evidence is already extremely weak for chiropractic care, adding in a control for the placebo effect would make the evidence even weaker. Another issue with these studies is for the most part, they only dealt with back pain. Many chiropractors claim to be able to treat all types of pain and bodily illnesses. Considering chiropractors pride themselves on being the "back specialists," if the studies indicate there's no evidence they can help with your back, what would be the probability they would be able to cure you high blood pressure by adjusting your C7?

But this doesn't mean it's completely disproven right? I mean there's still a chance it might work, so why not give it a try? No, don't give it a try, with the reason being the safety risks, some of which can be extremely dangerous. We'll go over these later in the book.

Practitioners of alternative medicine are able to make boisterous claims because of anecdotal evidence. You cannot prove or disprove that claim without a clinical study. When pharmaceutical companies want to get a drug approved to market, they have to run double blind, placebo controlled studies or else the FDA won't even consider looking at the drug. A drug company could never just say "well we have 5 patients who took it and they feel great. Can we get approval?" It's possible the medication worked, but it's also possible that it was all placebo, not to mention all the possible side effects or issues associated with the medication that are unknown without long term studies. Without this same type of scrupulous criteria applied to chiropractics, they can make all types of beneficial health claims because they do not have to prove it. [10]

A systematic review was performed in 2003, as in a review the compiles multiple studies on chiropractics, and it found massage therapy to be more effective than chiropractic care for back pain. It's making more sense to have that massage therapist in your office now. [11]

John Morrison

CHAPTER 5
Chiropractic Schooling

In the United States chiropractors are called "doctors." This is almost a fallacy though, and can distort someone's understanding of what it actually took to get that title. Whenever we hear the word "doctor," we immediately think of someone who did extremely well during their undergrad years in college and was able to get into one of the extremely competitive medical schools. They then went through at least an additional eight years of schooling, possibly more, to get their title as a medical doctor. Or we may think of a college professor, who also had to go through extensive schooling and write a dissertation in order to be awarded a PhD in their field of study. Chiropractic school is a little different.

All chiropractic schools in the United States have very little criteria to get in. While some applicants possess bachelor's degrees, chiropractic schools do not require them for admission. You are required to have at least 90 hours worth of college credit, and the schools do have a minimum GPA of at least 2.75; that's about where the criteria ends though. All Palmer College of Chiropractics, located in Iowa, Florida, Wisconsin, and California have a 100% acceptance rate. Parker University in Texas has a 100% acceptance rate. Logan University in Missouri has a 100% acceptance rate. Noticing a pattern here? Have you ever heard of a medical school, or even an undergraduate institution having a 100% acceptance rate? There are some community colleges that don't even have a 100% acceptance rate! I want you to truly think about what a "100%" acceptance rate means. Any Moe, Curly, or Larry can get into their school so as long as they have some college experience or a bachelor's degree, and have gotten by with B's and C's. No MCAT type entrance exam, no wait lists, nothing. So as long as you have some college experience, a pulse, and can pay for their school, they will let you in. Is this who you want adjusting your back or neck, and providing you with potentially life changing medical therapy? [12]

And I want you to think about something; if any student can get in, then we have to assume that the actual schooling when they get there cannot be too difficult, or else they would lose most of their students to poor grades. While I have no conclusive evidence, I would assume they most likely have to "water down" the schooling, to allow more of their students to pass, and thus obtain higher test scores and higher graduation rates. They cannot afford to lose the students who come to their schools to poor test grades. Considering tuition for many schools comes out to around $32,000 a year, this would result in far too much lost money for the school. [13]

CHAPTER 6
Potential Harm of Chiropractic Treatment

You may still be holding out for chiropractic treatment, in the hopes it might work for you. You think to yourself, what's the harm of going a couple times, it might work right? Well there actually is a great deal of potential harm, particularly if the chiropractor is adjusting your neck. I really wish someone shared this information with me before I went to the chiropractor.

The evidence suggests over half of all patients who visit chiropractors have mild to moderate adverse effects for a few days after being adjusted. Most likely this is because parts of the body are being manipulated that shouldn't be, and thus the body has to heal itself. Then there's the not so pretty fact that hundreds of cases have been reported where patients have been permanently damaged after chiropractic treatment, up to and including death. Dramatic complications are reported with alarming regularity in chiropractics. And though we have all this documented evidence, a bigger issue is many patients may sustain some form of injury after chiropractic adjustment, and just quit going to their chiropractor without reporting it to an advisory board. Considering this, there are an exponentially larger number of complications related to chiropractics that go unreported. [14]

Getting your neck adjusted appears to be the most dangerous treatment method. The quick, sharp thrusts used in these adjustments can cause tears in the artery walls of the neck. Blood clots can form at the site of the tear, which can end up breaking free, blocking a blood vessel in the brain and ultimately causing a stroke. Effects from strokes include a whole range of neurological problems, and can result in death. And older clients aren't the only ones at risk, as these neck adjustments can cause strokes in young people as well. [15]

Katie May had everything going for her. She was a model for Playboy, had a huge following on Instagram and Snapchat and was only 34 years old, with many years left to live. She was performing a photoshoot and started feeling a pain in her neck. Instead of going to a regular doctor, she decided to go to a chiropractor to help her with this issue. She may have seen an ad like the one on the next page, which are very common among chiropractors.

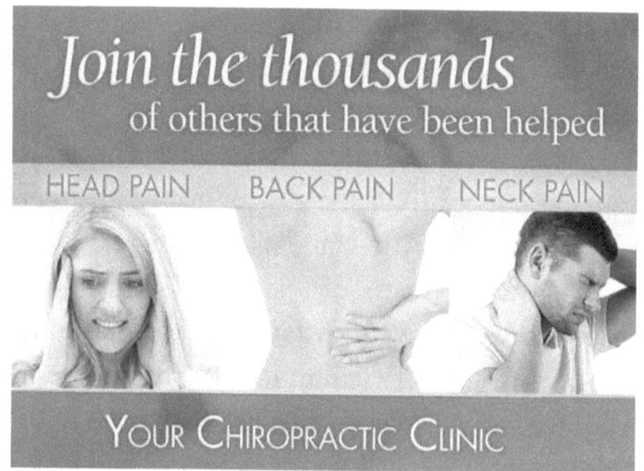

The same evening she went to the chiropractor, she collapsed and was rushed to the hospital. She died three days later. The autopsy report revealed she died from "a blunt force injury during a neck manipulation by [a] chiropractor." The injury caused a tear in her artery, cutting off blood flow to her brain, which ended up causing her death. [16]

In November 2014, 30 year old Jeremy Youngblood of Ada, Oklahoma visited a chiropractor. Within minutes of receiving a chiropractic adjustment on his neck, Jeremy collapsed onto the floor. Instead of calling 911, the clinic called Jeremy's father to come get him. His father rushed him to the hospital, where he laid for six hours before dying. The autopsy report revealed Jeremy died of, "acute cerebellar infarction due to manipulation of the neck." In layman's terms, this indicates Jeremy died of a stroke, just like the previous victim Katie May. [17]

These two examples prove that chiropractic treatment, especially in the case of neck adjustments, can prove deadly. And while all complications don't result in death, there can still be serious health consequences. Take for instance a case study in the National Institute of Health of a 38 year old female school teacher who received a neck adjustment from a chiropractor. She had no previous medical history, yet a short time after receiving a chiropractic neck adjustment she started experiencing, "headache, nausea, vomiting, blurred vision, diplopia, dizziness, and ataxia." Ataxia is a neurological disorder with symptoms that mimic someone who is drunk including slurred speech and difficulty walking. She slowly began losing consciousness and when admitted to the hospital, couldn't follow basic commands. An operation called a "ventriculostomy" had to be performed, which is where they create a hole in the skull to drain blood and/or spinal fluid. The patient was discharged after 12 days, but still had "residual left-sided facial weakness and impaired sensation" when she left. The case study found this patient had a "vertebral artery aneurysm" which caused a stroke. [18]

These are just a few of the hundreds of reported cases of serious complications from chiropractic treatment. Considering the cases just mentioned, as well as the many more reported and unreported cases of serious injury or death from chiropractic treatment, is it really worth the risk/reward to go to a chiropractor and get adjusted? They may help you, but they also may seriously injure or kill you. And considering the large scale studies prove that they provide no advantage over conventional medical treatments, there is no reason to go to a chiropractor, even for a minor issue.

CHAPTER 7
Chiropractors Replacing Doctors

A big issue with chiropractics is patients think they are going to a qualified medical professional, when in actuality they are going to a provider who is trained in pseudoscience. These providers are trained in "vertebral subluxation," as in restoring the nervous system through the spine, and not in traditional medicine. So patients with serious medical conditions can end up getting misdiagnosed and treated with "vertebral subluxation," which delays highly needed medical intervention. Many chiropractors have started portraying themselves as "family doctors," in an effort to replace a traditional primary care provider. Ads like the one on the next page are common among those in chiropractics:

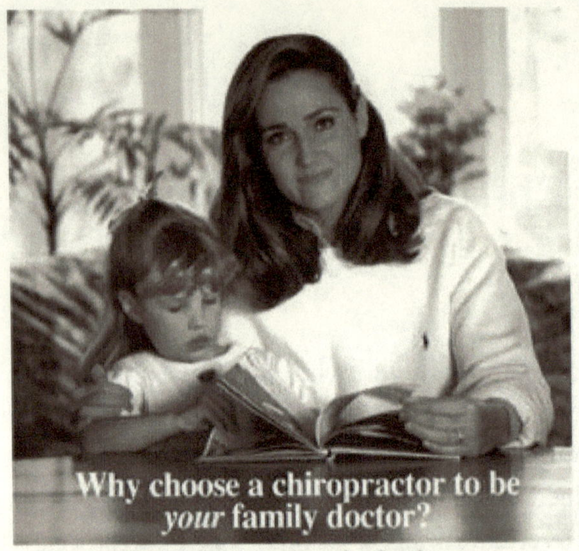

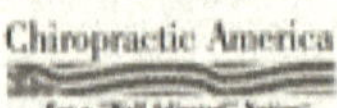

There is a chiropractor in my home state of North Carolina who runs radio ads constantly advertising a seminar. He claims to be able to fix thyroid issues, diabetes, and a host of other problems with a special diet that doctors "don't test for." And that by coming to his seminar and giving him your money, he will be able cure you. There are many other chiropractors, whether it be online or at their own offices, giving out similar health advice. What gives any of these chiropractors the qualifications to claim they can treat all your health ailments like a primary care doctor? That's like a gynecologist claiming he can fix your shoulder.

In 2003 an anesthesiologist (MD) by the name of John Kinsinger wanted to see if chiropractors really had the medical knowledge they claimed to have. He performed a small, self-run experiment on whether or not chiropractors would be able to make proper medical diagnoses when presented with symptoms of serious medical conditions. He visited nine chiropractors during the study, and all the symptoms John brought up were fake, as he had no serious medical conditions. Here are some of those cases.

At the first provider John visited, he posed as an uninsured real estate agent suffering from erectile dysfunction. Within a few minutes of examining his back, John was told she had located "a spinal abnormality that was very likely the source of [his] problem." John asked if she would like to examine his genitals, but was told it was not necessary. John shaved his beard, and visited this same chiropractor six months later. This time he posed as an uninsured construction worker with chest pain that radiated into his left shoulder and upper arm. These are classic symptoms of limited blood flow to the heart, which puts John at a high risk for a heart attack. While she did listen to John's heart, she concluded his ribs were out of alignment, and getting them back to a normal range of motion would improve his condition.

At the second chiropractor, John stated he had recently helped a friend move furniture and hurt his back. Before the visit John had a full x-ray of his back evaluated by a radiologist (MD), who determined it looked completely fine with no abnormalities. John brought these films with him to show the chiropractor, not mentioning they were examined previously. During his visit, the chiropractor's assistant performed a series of tests, asking John if he felt pain anywhere she touched him. He stated he wasn't having much pain. The chiropractor proceeded to exam his spine and, with a sense of urgency, stated John needed a full spinal x-ray at his office. The chiropractor said he had located issues on the x-ray films John had brought in, and wanted John to return the next day for a counseling session to discuss a treatment plan. John did not return.

At the third chiropractor, John posed as an uninsured construction worker with right lower abdominal pain associated with nausea, a common symptom of appendicitis. He told the provider the pain had started two days prior. The chiropractor stated there was a "shift," as he felt the thoracic region of John's back. He brought up a "pinched nerve" and "muscle spasms," and stated there was a virus going around that John could have caught. He then offered John a "little adjustment," which John declined and said he had to think about. This chiropractor did not feel John's abdomen, check him for a fever, or ask about prior surgical history in the abdominal region.

At the fourth chiropractor, John walked in presenting the same abdominal symptoms. This time, the young chiropractor asked John if he ever had his appendix removed, which John denied. The chiropractor stated appendicitis was a possibility, but wanted to check him with an exam. He found John's right leg to be shorter than his left, and that because John placed his wallet in his back right pocket, it was causing a buildup of lactic acid in his stomach leading to a "side stitch." He then performed a spinal x-ray on John, and found a narrowed disc space in John's lower spine. The chiropractor stated John's pain could be due to a pinched nerve in this narrowed disc space. He suggested John try chiropractic treatment, and if his condition didn't improve within a couple days, to go get an MD's evaluation for possible appendicitis.

While this may seem like practical advice, a two

day window could mean death for someone with actual appendicitis. [19] While this is a relatively small scale study, it does show how ill-equipped chiropractors are to handle serious medical conditions. Unfortunately there aren't any large scale studies currently available for this issue, as it would get a little tricky getting so many undercover patients. However there is more evidence provided in the next chapter performed by a major news outlet.

CHAPTER 8

Marketing to Children and Infants

In an effort to increase their clientele, many chiropractors have begun marketing treatment to children and infants, as young as just a few days old. Ads like the one below are quite common (I have marked out all personal information on ad for privacy reasons):

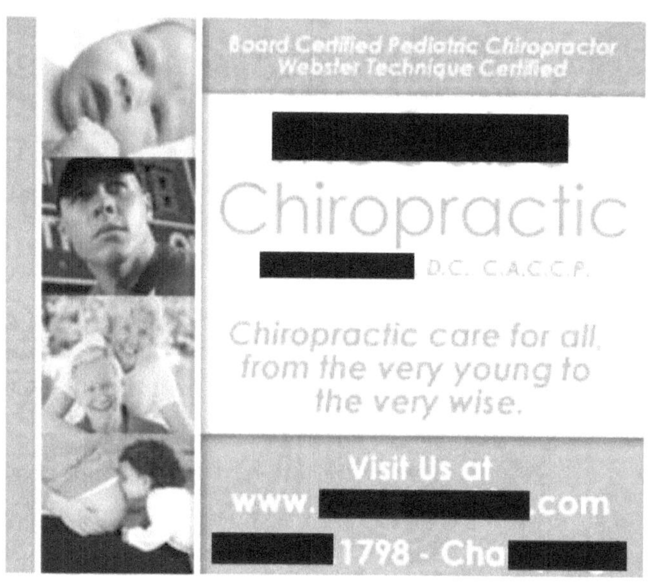

Notice there is a picture of a newborn baby at the top, and the ad says "from the very young to the very wise." Sherman College of Chiropractic in Boiling Springs, SC lists this on their website:

> "We know, for example, that specific adjustments can help the body correct subluxations. We also know that children and even infants benefit from gentle adjustments performed by doctors of chiropractic. But what about animals? Many students new to the field of chiropractic might not know that our furry friends also benefit from the care of a trained chiropractor." [20]

So not only should you bring your two day old infant to your local chiropractor to have their back cracked, you should bring your rabbit too! Unfortunately, like many other areas of chiropractics, there have not been many studies on if chiropractic treatment works for infants. One of the few studies performed evaluated 100 infants who were treated with chiropractic therapy for colic. Colic is basically uncontrolled crying in infants, and its cause is unknown. The study found "chiropractic spinal manipulation is no more effective than placebo in the treatment of infantile colic." [21]

Considering there is no reliable evidence chiropractic therapy works for infants, and the few studies that have been performed state it works no better than placebo, you would think chiropractors would be a little hesitate about cracking infants backs. However this has not stopped them. While I don't have an exact number in the United States, a survey of 1200 chiropractors in Canada found almost all treated patients younger than 18 years old. [22]

There was a famous 20/20 investigation on ABC done in the early 90's. During the investigation, the crew found a number of chiropractors who stated on their advertisements they treated infants. They brought an infant named Blake to nine of these chiropractors with a hidden camera. Blake had been diagnosed by a pediatrician (MD) with an ear infection, a problem that could be treated with antibiotics and rest and relaxation. All nine of the chiropractors found a problem with the baby, and care was recommended ranging from several weeks to a whole lifetime. The alarming part of this segment was the dichotomy in treatment methods from all visited chiropractors. While I'm sure this does sometimes occur in traditional medicine, for the most part, it is rare. If your infant has an ear infection and you go to nine different ENT's, most likely all nine will diagnosis your infant with an ear infection and provide an antibiotic; this wasn't the case with the nine chiropractors videotaped. You'd have to go to hundreds of ENT's before you found an outlier who treated such a well-known, common issue as an ear infection with something other than an antibiotic and rest and relaxation.

The first chiropractor found a "misalignment between the second and third bones in his neck." The second chiropractor found a misalignment "on the right side of his neck between the first and second bones." The third performed a muscle test and found "weakness in the adrenal glands." The fourth stated subluxation, as in a misalignment of the spine, was occurring because one of the baby's legs was shorter than the other. The fifth asked the boy's mother to touch him on the shoulder, while the chiropractor pulled on the mother's arm, as this was his method of diagnosis. The six did a similar test; he pulled on the mother's leg while the infant, Blake, laid on her back. He diagnosed Blake with "jamming of the occiput" and corrected it by lifting Blake's occiput with his thumbs (the occiput is the lower back part of the skull). He also said Blake "needed work on his immune system."

The 20/20 program ran another segment visiting eight chiropractors in Wisconsin. They had a five year old boy who had been diagnosed with a severe ear infection. And while all eight chiropractors did find problems with the boy's ear, they differed in their method of treatment. One chiropractor diagnosed the boy with a pinched nerve in his neck. Another said his right leg was shorter than his left. Another said his left leg was shorter than his right. One chiropractor said the boy had a zinc deficiency. Another chiropractor said the boy's ear problem stemmed from food sensitivities, and told him to stop eating corn, cow's milk, and white flour. Another said the boy had a subluxation in the top part of his spine. And one more chiropractor said it wasn't an ear problem at all, but instead scoliosis (which was disputed by a pediatrician and radiologist). [23]

What these findings show is chiropractors are not medical doctors, and do not receive the same training. The curriculum at chiropractic schools is much different, and focuses on the "vertebral subluxation" that was mentioned before. This training does not allow chiropractors to properly diagnosis medical issues, and unlike conventional medicine, is obviously very subjective to the provider. We have the same condition brought in, and a different treatment method brought about by each provider. This is extremely rare in traditional medicine, and further validates the thesis that chiropractic theory is a hoax.

CHAPTER 9
Why Does Insurance Pay For Chiropractic Treatment

This is an interesting topic. If chiropractic treatment is nothing more than the placebo effect and could actually harm patients, why are insurance companies covering the charge and paying for it? Well it wasn't always this way. In fact for many years, insurance companies had nothing to do with chiropractic treatment. But along comes big government and their overreaching arm.

Originally, only states with chiropractic schools required insurance companies to cover chiropractic medicine. Chiropractic schools have lobbyist, and they convinced state government officials that not only is chiropractic medicine helpful, but their schools would bring money to the state. And when money is involved, poor choices can be made.

Soon, the federal government became involved. Senator Orrin Hatch out of Utah was a big proponent of chiropractic medicine. He used his power to push laws into place requiring many more states and insurance companies to cover chiropractic medicine, treating it the same as conventional medicine. Usually when someone is such a big proponent of something, such as Orrin Hatch was, there is good reason behind it. Orrin has two daughters who both married chiropractic doctors. And their lives, and paychecks, ended up improving greatly after insurance started paying out chiropractic claims.

Chiropractic colleges and lobbyist still have a lot of power. Most recently in 2017 they pushed a bill through the state of Wisconsin which allowed chiropractors to "perform physical exams on high school and 2 year UW college student athletes." [24]

CHAPTER 10
Why Does Chiropractic Treatment Work For Some People

The reason chiropractic treatment works for some people is the same reason other types of disproven alternative medicine works for some people. Firstly, you are provided one on one time with the provider. Many chiropractors have full one hour appointments with their clients where they talk with them about their life. Here you have a commanding medical professional, usually in a white coat, with their doctorate hanging on the wall. They begin telling you the exact reason why you have pain and how they will certainly be able to help you. They then give you individualized, one on one therapy, going over any part of your body that hurts you. They form a relationship with you, learning about your personal life and your past. Many chiropractors also incorporate massage therapy into their practice. So take into account a commanding "doctor" telling you they will fix you, the placebo effect, a nice massage, and a little bit of time, and many issues will go away on their own naturally.

Compare this to many doctor's offices nowadays which have become an insurance number factory. You're rushed during your whole appointment, given maybe 10 minutes to talk to the doctor if you're lucky, and then sent to a pharmacy to pick up some pills. It's a completely different experience. And while the doctor and those pills may help you, people want more. Many people enjoy talking about themselves and they want someone who will listen to them. And a chiropractor usually does just that, while providing one on one treatment. This all further enhances the placebo effect.

Conclusion

I hope you now fully understand the science behind chiropractics, and why going to one (or becoming one) would be a complete waste of your time and money, and a potential risk to your health. While some alternative medicine may turn out to be true, you must remain a little skeptical and make sure the science behind it is sound and there are studies which prove it. Anecdotal evidence is weak, and should never be used to make serious medical decisions. I encourage you to look at the references provided and do more research on the subject yourself. You'll see that the facts stated in this book are true and chiropractors cannot back up the claims they profess. Money is the root of all evil, and I feel much of chiropractic medicine can be linked to it, much the same other types of alternative medicine can be linked to money. If someone will pay for a service, someone else will provide it.

If you enjoyed this book, please leave a 5 star review on Amazon. It is greatly appreciated! The link below will take you right to the review page:

<u>fastlink.xyz/chiro</u>

If you have any questions regarding this book, feel free to email me at <u>john@unknownwealth.com</u>.

If you enjoyed this book, you may also like…

Evolution's Final Days

The Mounting Evidence Disproving the Theory of Evolution

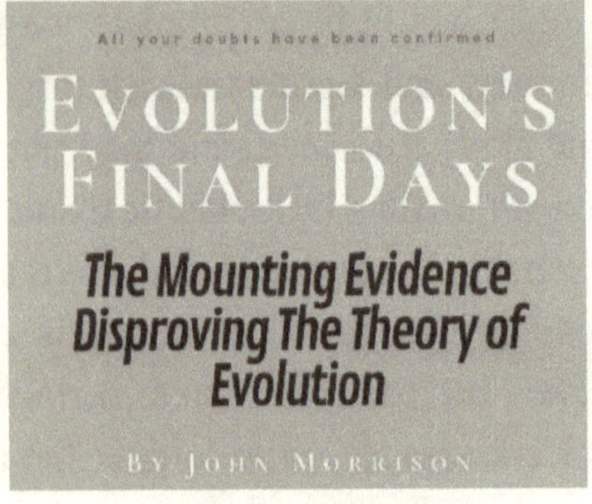

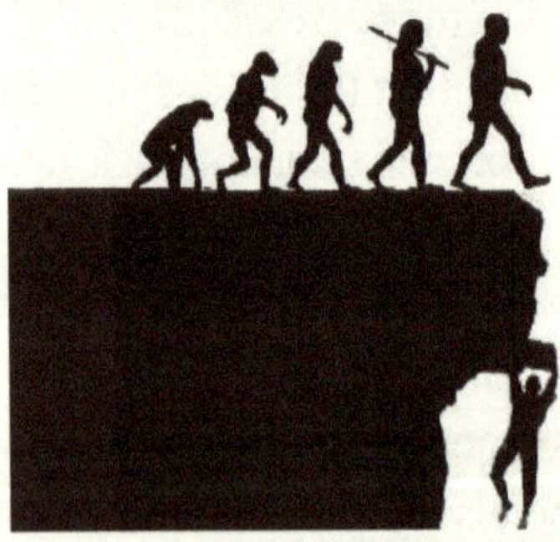

Shortened Link to Amazon Page: **fastlink.xyz/efd**

In this groundbreaking book, author John Morrison brings to light new evidence which puts many holes in the theory of evolution. Going over the fossil record, the laws of the universe, and biochemistry, John proves to readers the theory of evolution could have never happened as claimed. Find out more at the link above!

REFERENCES

[1]https://www.myovision.com/scanvision.html

[2]https://www.chirobase.org/05RB/palmer_1910.pdf

[3]https://en.wikipedia.org/wiki/Chiropractic#History

[4]https://en.wikipedia.org/wiki/Daniel_David_Palme
r#Discovery_of_chiropractic

[5]https://www.chiropractic.org.nz/about-
chiropractic/vertebral-subluxation/

[6]https://lifewest.edu/about/about-chiropractic/

[7]https://www.ncbi.nlm.nih.gov/pmc/articles/PMC27
94701/

[8]https://www.quackwatch.org/01QuackeryRelatedT
opics/chirosub.html

[9]https://www.ncbi.nlm.nih.gov/pubmed/9112710

[10]https://www.ncbi.nlm.nih.gov/pmc/articles/PMC1
447290/

[11]https://annals.org/aim/article-
abstract/716463/review-evidence-effectiveness-safety-
cost-acupuncture-massage-therapy-spinal-
manipulation?year=2003

[12a]https://www.google.com/search?q=palmer+colle
ge+of+chiropractic+acceptance+rate&rlz=1C1NHXL
_enUS825US825&oq=palmer+college&aqs=chrome.
2.0j69i57j35i39l2j0l2.3718j0j4&sourceid=chrome&ie
=UTF-8

[12b]https://www.petersons.com/college-
search/logan-university-college-of-chiropractic-
000_10001744.aspx

[12c]https://www.niche.com/colleges/parker-
university/

[12d]https://www.life.edu/academic-pages/chiropractic/academic-pageschiropracticadmission-requirements/

[13]https://www.sherman.edu/knowledge-base/what-is-the-cost-of-tuition/

[14]https://www.ncbi.nlm.nih.gov/pmc/articles/PMC1447290/

[15]https://healthblog.uofmhealth.org/wellness-prevention/chiropractic-neck-manipulation-and-stroke-whats-risk

[16]https://health.spectator.co.uk/the-evidence-shows-that-chiropractors-do-more-harm-than-good/

[17]https://kfor.com/2014/11/03/30-year-old-dies-after-visit-to-the-chiropractor/

[18]https://www.ncbi.nlm.nih.gov/pmc/articles/PMC4264725/

[19]https://www.quackwatch.org/01QuackeryRelatedTopics/chiroinv.html

[20]https://www.sherman.edu/category/chiropractic-profession/

[21]https://www.ncbi.nlm.nih.gov/pubmed/11159288

[22]https://www.ncbi.nlm.nih.gov/pmc/articles/PMC2794701/

[23]https://www.chirobase.org/02Research/chiroinv.html

[24]http://legis.wisconsin.gov/assembly/44/kolste/media/1102/chiropractic-bill-shows-the-power-of-lobbyists-and-money-in-state-government.pdf

www.ingramcontent.com/pod-product-compliance
Lightning Source LLC
Chambersburg PA
CBHW051415250726
48655CB00003B/1056